Instant Baby Food

Linda McDonald is also author of:

Baby's Recipe Book
Ice Cream, Sherbet, and Ices
Contact Lenses: How to Wear Them Successfully
Everything You Need to Know About Babies
The Joy of Breastfeeding

Instant Baby Food

Linda McDonald

Illustrations by Vicki Erickson

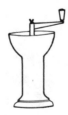

Oaklawn Press
283 South Lake Avenue
Pasadena, California 91101
1975

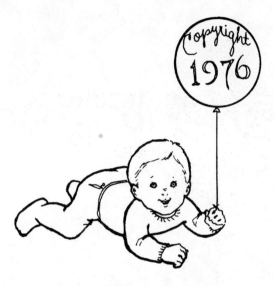

Library of Congress Cataloging in Publication Data

McDonald, Linda.
    Instant baby food.

    Includes index.
        1. Cookery (Baby foods)   2. Infants—Nutrition.
I. Title.
TX740.M146   641.5'622   75-27760
ISBN 0-916198-01-4
Illustrations by Vicki Erickson

Copyright © 1975, by Linda McDonald
First Edition 1975
Revised Edition Copyright © 1976 by Linda McDonald
Ninth printing: April 1981

Published by Oaklawn Press, Inc.
283 South Lake Avenue, Pasadena, California 91101

Printed in the United States of America

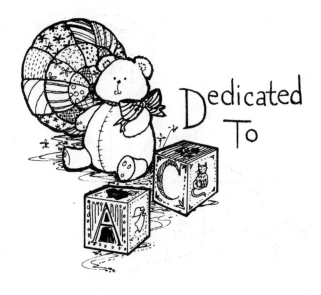

Dedicated
To

mothers everywhere

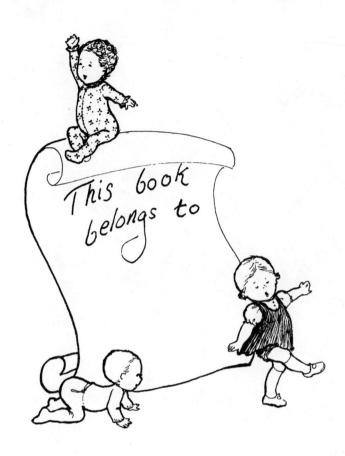

This book
belongs to

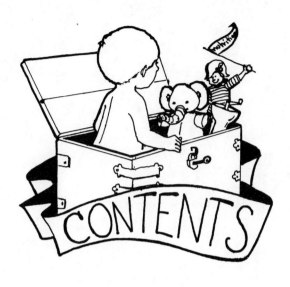

CONTENTS

Introduction to the Second Edition

Paul Murray Fleiss, M.D., Fellow of the American Academy of Pediatrics, is in the private practice of pediatrics in Hollywood, California. He is assistant clinical professor of pediatrics at the School of Medicine, University of Southern California, and attending staff member in pediatrics at Los Angeles Children's Hospital, Cedars-Sinai Medical Center, Hollywood Presbyterian Medical Center, and the Los Angeles County - University of Southern California Medical Center. Dr. Fleiss and his wife, Elissa, have never purchased a jar of commercially prepared baby food or infant formula for any of their five children.

In *Instant Baby Food*, the fact has been brought out that "Solid foods, when started too early, are nutritionally inferior to milk." The ideal food for infants is breast milk. All other milk or semi-solids are deficient in many of the hundreds of natural ingredients found in mothers' milk. Semi-solid foods may become part of the infant's diet at four to six months and reach about twenty-five percent of the infant's diet between six to twelve months of life.

For centuries the nourishment of infants and children and the preparation of their food has been the responsibility of their parents. The introduction of commercially prepared infant foods in the first half of the twentieth century took the preparation of baby food out of mothers' hands. The early, rapid acceptance of processed infant foods could be attributed to several factors—chiefly convenience and novelty. Advertising through various media has promoted the use of commercially prepared baby foods world-wide into every culture and every economic level.

Baby foods have become big business. Much money and effort go into promoting these foods, making them desirable to mothers everywhere. Sugar and salt are necessary to processing. While sugar and salt may appeal to mothers' tastes, neither is necessary for infant nutrition—indeed, the long range harmful effects of excess salt and sugar have not been determined. Artificial ingredients in commercial baby foods have been used to enhance attractiveness, and chemicals such as monosodium glutamate have been used to boost flavor.

Sodium nitrite and other preservatives were once used to prolong shelf-life. These substances have nothing to do with infant nutrition. Recent consumer pressure has led the industry to remove many of these questionably dangerous additives once present in commercial baby foods. However, a few objectionable additives still remain and probably always will.

Commercial baby food is expensive. The cost is approximately seven to eight times as much as fresh food prepared at home. To illustrate, fresh bananas can be purchased for 20¢ to 25¢ per pound while a jar of bananas costs about $1.80 to $2.00 per pound. Nutritionally much is lost in processing the fruit. A jar of bananas is composed of 30% bananas: Water, sugar, tapioca and filler make up the remaining 70%. Home-prepared fruit can be 100% pure, nutritious food.

Several things deserving of additional comment are brought out in Linda McDonald's book. She has cautioned that certain foods should be avoided because they are rich in calories but contain very little food value. Sugar adds unnecessary extra calories to infant foods. Too many calories consumed in early life lead to an obese infant, and perhaps to an obese child and adult. Babies' tastes can become accustomed to the excessive, artificial sweetness of food; and they may soon prefer sugar to the natural sweetness of fresh foods. Salt is another questionable ingredient of baby food. Too much salt in an infant's diet may have implications in the development of high blood pressure and heart failure in adult life.

In *Instant Baby Food*, none of Mrs. McDonald's recipes contain sugar, salt, artificial flavorings, colorings, processed foods or processed meats. Her selections, containing natural foods and natural sugar from ripe fruits, show that preparing nutritious food for one's infant is safe and economical.

It is possible for parents, with love and creativity, to nurture their infants with home-prepared food; and in doing so, parents and child will experience a great deal of pleasure at the same time. *Instant Baby Food* will tell you how.

Instant Baby Food

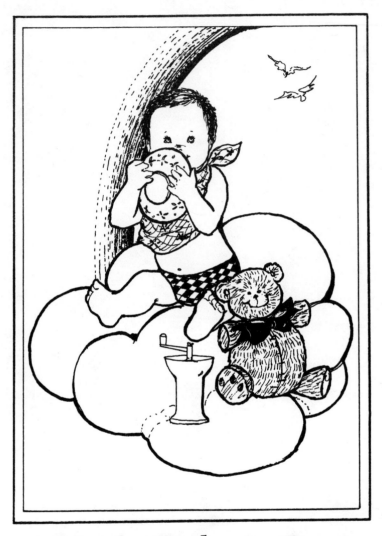

1. Your Baby's First Solid Food

When to start a baby on solid food is determined by several factors. Physical development, readiness and age are among them. Your doctor is best able to make this decision and to help you calculate the amount of food needed on the basis of these factors.

Babies differ widely and what works well for one may not apply to another. Your baby is an individual. He develops somewhat differently from every other baby so don't coax or force him to eat if he doesn't accept the food readily.

Another thing to keep in mind is that it takes many months for the tongue reflex to be fully developed in infants to the point where food is easily pushed to the back of the mouth. So if the baby resists by clamping his mouth shut, turning his head away, or spitting the food back out, it's just his way of telling you that he is not quite ready for solids.

Take his word for it; don't push, he will gradually learn to eat well. Baby knows instinctively when he is ready to eat and also how much he needs and what his digestion can handle.

Should any difficulty arise in feeding your baby it is best to get in touch with the doctor so he can observe your baby's development and make note of any problems. Sometimes foods may have to be taken out of the diet and others added to it. This will depend upon baby's digestion and progress. With just a little guidance your doctor can make things happy and convenient for all.

What to Feed Your Baby

When your baby is the right age your doctor will provide you with a list of foods to feed. The diet sheet he gives you should be your guide to using this book. Refer to the appropriate chapter for instructions on how to prepare each food on your diet sheet.

With the help of your baby food grinder you will be able to serve fresh food, instantly, at each meal, instead of relying on foods that may take hours of your time to prepare specially. All you have to do is moisten the freshly ground food with a little milk or some other liquid until it reaches just the right consistency.

Some doctors start babies on bananas or applesauce. Both of these foods have a pleasantly sweet flavor which most babies like and readily digest. Other doctors recommend cereal as the first solid. The disadvantage of starting with cereal is that babies find it unappetizing. Whatever the preference, don't offer too many foods too quickly; this may cause sudden upsets.

Feeding your baby pureed leftovers is not recommended. Such foods are too likely to be inferior due to vitamin deterioration and bacterial growth. This is a very good reason not to make baby food ahead of time either, or to store it for future use.

Milk Before Solids

Solid foods, when started too early, are nutritionally inferior to milk. When you offer milk, first, you can be assured your baby is getting the best food first. When you offer milk first it also helps to take the edge off baby's appetite. When a baby is too hungry he is not too eager to experiment with new foods. After you have gone along for a month or two with milk first, try the solid food first; then end the meal with milk or a little fruit juice.

How to Feed Solids

A baby, who has been used to sucking only, will find solids a little bewildering. The feel of a spoon is quite different from the feel of a soft nipple. So don't be surprised, on the first time, if your baby pushes the spoonful of food onto his chin. If he doesn't do that he is more than likely to make a sucking motion that will spread the food in different directions.

Be patient and start over. It won't be long before he catches on. For the first few days it is recommended that you hold the baby in your lap, tilting him back ever so slightly as you offer the food. This technique will help the food go down a little easier. Also, most babies prefer being fed with a plastic spoon because it is softer and lighter than a silver spoon. A plastic spoon is easier on gums too and does not feel hot or cold.

How Much to Feed

When you're first beginning solids it's best to give your baby just a taste for the first few days. Most doctors recommend starting with a teaspoonful or less of food. You may even want to begin with as little as a quarter-teaspoonful until he indicates to you that he'd like more. This can gradually be worked up to two or three tablespoonfuls in a week or two.

Introducing New Foods

The best way to acquaint baby with new foods is to do it so gradually he hardly knows it's happening at all. Introduce them one at a time, giving only a quarter-teaspoonful of the new food each day. The reason for this is to avoid a possible allergic reaction. If the new food is agreeable you can increase the amount little by little until baby is getting whatever he can handle.

Doctors usually recommend waiting at least four to seven days before introducing a new food. They also advise using a "single food." This means a single fruit, a single vegetable, a single cereal and so forth.

Don't add anything at all to the bananas, carrots, peas or cereal. When you mix a previously offered food with pudding, stew or mixed-grain cereals it becomes exceedingly complex, if there's an allergic reaction, to determine if the baby is sensitive to eggs, milk products or wheat and other cereals. "Mixed foods" are liable to contain any of these ingredients. Therefore, it is best not to let the baby get acquainted with too many foods too soon.

Single Foods	*Mixed Foods*
Applesauce	Breads
Bananas	Omelets
Carrots	Soups
Peas	Stews
Squash	Puddings
Beef	Cereals

Finger Foods for Munching

Some time in the second half of the first year, when baby's teeth begin to come through, he will chew on everything — his toys, the side of his playpen, his fingers. When he starts to do this it's time to let him know that he can chew food.

Finger foods are given to babies for several reasons. They help ease his way through the discomforts of teething; they help to develop finger control, and muscular coordination; and they familiarize the baby with coarser foods.

Don't count on a baby getting his nourishment from finger foods. They're meant just for gnawing and development, as he is not yet equipped with molars to grind up food that will easily go down.

At first try offering a piece of hard toast. Then give him a bone with just a tiny bit of meat on it. Just be sure to remove any gristle so there is nothing for the baby to choke on. Most babies love to work over a chicken leg, sucking and chewing on its goodness.

Raw apple, banana, pear, carrot and celery sticks are also good. Some mothers even like to chill these foods first because their coolness helps soothe tingling bare gums.

Good eating habits should start early so always offer a baby nourishing foods to munch on. They are the only foods that supply the essential nutrients for health and growth. Avoid sweet teething biscuits, cakes and cookies, which certainly are not foods that build muscle, bones, blood and sound teeth.

Changing Over to Junior Dinners

If all along you have been giving baby foods prepared in a baby food grinder then you will probably experience no difficulty in changing over to coarser foods. A baby who has been getting freshly ground food all along is less likely to balk at accepting food in a more adult form.

To start on a more grown-up diet use either or both of the following plans. Use vegetables or fruits as usual and then press them through the food grinder, but add some larger pieces to the mixture. Or, let him pick up these bigger pieces by himself if he wishes.

When mixing foods of different textures for the first time you will want to use more of the ground food and perhaps reduce the size of the chopped pieces. Gradually decrease the ground portion as the baby can handle it.

Or, you can use another method. Give the baby pieces of food: bits of meat, a cooked vegetable such as carrots or string beans, or pieces of raw fruit such as peeled apples, pears, bananas, or wedges of cheese. Let him chew off whatever he can handle.

For the first two years use only fruits that you can wash or peel. Excessive amounts of dried fruits may cause loose bowels whereas fresh fruits may do the opposite. Also note that as a baby is learning to manage more adult foods, chunks of imperfectly digested food may appear in his bowel movements.

If you change to coarser foods or bits of foods gradually it won't be long before you will be able to feed him what you prepare for the rest of the family. If family meals are kept simple, without highly spiced dishes, rich pastries, or sweet fatty foods, you should not have to make any special plans for the baby. The simpler the foods the better. A diet selected from the basic food groups, simply prepared, can be enjoyed by the entire family.

How to Make Foods Palatable

Color, taste and texture play an important role in making your baby's food palatable. As babies get older they become quite sensitive to color in their food, so at mealtime do whatever you can to add a spark of interest.

Carrots, squash, peas, green beans and strawberries all help to perk up appetites. A sunny spot in the kitchen and bright mugs and place mats also help to liven up the color scheme.

If babies and young children are given a choice they will always favor foods with mild, delicate flavors. As you probably may have noticed strong flavored or unpleasant tasting foods are less popular than others. For example, broccoli, brussels sprouts and cauliflower are not as popular as carrots, peas or squash.

It is best to remember to serve only one of the less popular vegetables at each mealtime. If you gradually let a baby encounter the less favorable food, or perhaps mix a little fruit with it, there is a greater chance he will feel more friendly toward it later on. Go slowly and do not force him. After a month or two you may find him enjoying it along with his regular food.

Babies are quite sensitive to the texture in foods and will notice the difference between soft, creamy foods, crisp raw fruits and buttery pieces of crunchy toast.

A good way to hold interest at mealtime is to offer one crunchy food and one soft food. Chewy foods, like pieces of cooked meat and some bread crusts, can be a little hard to handle, so only offer them occasionally.

Also avoid mixing too many foods together. Foods that have been mixed with other foods on the plate are not very palatable, either, so try to serve separate mounds of each food.

When serving any main dish encourage toddlers to consume the cooking liquids; some of the nutritive value is retained here.

Baby's Seasonings and Sweeteners

There is really no need to add seasonings or sweeteners to baby's food. Tests have shown that babies have absolutely no taste discrimination between salted and unsalted food.

Natural food has enough salt to suit baby's taste and to meet his physiological needs for sodium. There is no need to add salt to his food. When older babies are introduced to butter use the unsalted variety.

When the time comes to give Junior Dinners and Toddler Meals there is no necessity to exclude foods which are moderately or normally spiced, since there is no evidence in the medical literature that such foods are harmful. Babies may or may not like the foods as seasoned for the family. If he doesn't, then he solves the problem for himself very nicely by simply refusing to eat them.

Ripe fruits will provide baby with all the natural sugar he needs, and when you are ready to serve puddings and custards you can fold in a little fresh ripened or canned fruit in place of sugar.

The Best Sweeteners

Apricots	Applesauce
Bananas	Plums
Pears	Berries
Figs	Peaches
Raisins	Papayas
Dates	Mangos
Prunes	Tropical fruits
Currants	Dried fruits

Foods to Avoid

There are certain foods that should be avoided or served less frequently than others because they are rich in calories but contain very little food value. They include any refined sweets, refined starches or excessively salty or fatty foods. These foods may temporarily satisfy a child's hunger but they are very low in vitamins, minerals and protein.

There are other foods that you will want to avoid too, not because they spoil baby's appetite for healthful foods but because he can swallow them the wrong way and choke.

Never give a baby nuts, corn, popcorn, raisins, peas or other hard foods the size of peas which could cause him to choke and possibly inhale bits into his lungs. The following foods should be avoided:

Cakes	Coffee
Cookies	Tea
Pastries	Carbonated drinks
Chocolate	Popcorn
Instant pudding	Pretzels
Diabetic products	Corn chips
Artificial sweeteners	Potato chips
Sweetened vegetables	Luncheon meats
Sweet pickles	Sausages
Sweet relishes	Rich sauces
Syrup	Rich gravies
Marmalade	Candied fruits
Jam	Ready-to-eat cereals
Jelly	Refined bread
Sugar	Chocolate pudding
Candy	Maraschino cherries

Drinking From a Cup

There is no fixed age for a baby to drink from a cup. Try to follow the baby's lead. If he appears to enjoy handling a cup then encourage it. He'll spill a lot and chew the lip at first, but with practice he'll learn to swallow smoothly.

Put in a little milk or juice, only a tablespoonful at first, and let him handle the cup himself. Gradually increase the liquid as he takes more from the cup.

Some babies will accept only water or juice from a cup — practically anything except milk. So if he happens to be reluctant to use a cup that has milk in it you may have to switch to juice.

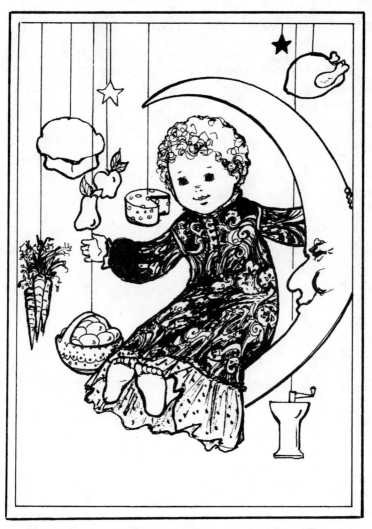

2. Foods From the Basic Food Groups

Foods from the basic food groups supply all of the essential nutrients for health and growth. These groups include milk and milk products, meats, vegetables and fruits, and breads and cereals. Every growing baby's diet, as he is ready to handle them, should include foods from each of these groups.

If meat is not a part of the diet use dry peas, beans, lentils, nuts, nut butters, peanuts and other vegetable proteins or meat substitutes.

If you find that your baby does not care for a food from a particular group then serve him another one from the same group that you know he likes. Babies, like grownups, have food preferences; so do not insist he eat foods that do not taste good to him.

One day he may eat a particular vegetable with great relish, while the next day he will turn it down. These preferences will vary from day to day. Children who are allowed to choose freely among nutritious foods will balance their own diets.

Babies' diets cannot be standardized because babies vary in their individual needs. Never try to make a baby fit a diet. The diet must be planned to fit the baby.

During the first year, your baby's diet should be supervised by your doctor. He is the one best qualified to advise you on your baby's nutritional requirements. He will tell you when to introduce the various food categories that will make up your baby's first-year menus.

Always use the four food groups as a guide for planning your baby's meals. The suggested servings that are given here are for children and grownups. You will only need a spoonful or two for baby. The food groups have been thoroughly covered because the successful use of your baby food grinder depends upon what you feed the entire family.

You will take small portions of fresh, frozen or canned foods that you have prepared for everyone else, and puree them in the food grinder to make healthful meals for the baby. Exactly how this is done will be discussed in greater detail in the chapters that follow.

Of course, there are other foods that will be used in family meals that are not included in these groups. They include sugars, butter, margarine, vegetable oils and other fats. These ingredients are often added to other foods during preparation or at the table.

The food guides that appear on the pages that follow sort foods into four groups on the basis of their similarity in nutrient content. Each group has a special contribution to make toward an adequate diet. Mothers who follow the guide will find it flexible enough in choosing foods for baby.

The foods in the four basic food groups are adaptable for persons of any age, to your family's food patterns and to baby's individual likes and dislikes. The food choices are wide enough to allow for variety in everyday foods, and to include family favorites, foods that fit the family budget, and foods that are available only in certain seasons.

Food from each group does not necessarily have to appear in each meal. The important thing is that the suggested number of servings from each of the groups be included sometime during the day. You can include additional foods from the four groups as well as other foods that are not listed here.

When your baby is old enough to handle Junior Dinners and Toddler Meals check the foods he eats against the following groups—milk and cottage cheese—meat and alternates such as beans, peas, lentils and eggs—carrots, squash, potatoes, sweet potatoes, green beans, peas, spinach, asparagus and beets—apples, apricots, bananas, pears, peaches, plums, pineapple, mangoes, papaya, prunes, orange, apple and other fruit juices—rice cereal, barley cereal, wheat cereal and oatmeal.

Milk and Milk Products

Milk is part of every baby's diet. If milk is not used for some reason substitute other calcium and protein containing foods.

Milk can also be offered in cooked dishes. Cheese and occasionally ice cream may replace part of the milk. A 1-inch cube of cheddar cheese may be used in place of ½ cup of milk; ½ cup cottage cheese for ⅓ cup milk; 2 tablespoons cream cheese for 1 tablespoon milk; or ½ cup ice cream for ¼ cup milk. Use any of the following:

Whole fluid milk	Cottage cheese
Concentrated milk	Cream cheese
Evaporated milk	Yogurt cheese
Buttermilk	Yogurt
Skim milk	Liquid yogurt
Dry milk	Soy milk
Cheese	Ice cream

Meat

Foods in the meat group are the primary source of protein in the diet. Plan two servings daily of meat, fish, poultry or eggs. Beans, peas, lentils, nuts and peanut butter may be used as alternates.

The following are approximately equal in the amount of protein they provide: 1 ounce of cooked lean meat, poultry, or fish; 1 egg; ½ cup cooked dried peas or beans; 2 tablespoons of peanut butter.

Count as a serving: 2 to 3 ounces of lean cooked meat, poultry, or fish; 2 eggs; 1 cup cooked dry beans, dry peas, or lentils; 4 tablespoons peanut butter. Choose from the following foods:

Beef	Fish
Veal	Beans
Lamb	Peas
Liver	Lentils
Poultry	Nuts
Eggs	Peanut Butter

Vegetables and Fruits

A citrus fruit, tomato or other good source of vitamin C should be eaten every day, and every other day a dark-green or deep-yellow vegetable for vitamin A.

Choose four or more servings every day. One-half cup of vegetable or fruit counts as one serving. Use other fruits and vegetables, including potatoes, to provide roughage, food energy and variety. The following fruits and vegetables are a good source of vitamin A.

Apricots	Mangos
Broccoli	Persimmons
Cantaloupe	Pumpkins
Carrots	Spinach
Chard	Sweet potatoes
Collards	Turnip greens
Cress	Winter squash
Kale	

The following list of fruits and vegetables shows some of the sources of vitamin C:

Good Sources	*Fair Sources*
Grapefruit	Tomatoes
Oranges	Cabbage
Strawberries	Melons
Cantaloupe	Tangerines
Green peppers	Cress
Sweet red peppers	Mustard greens
Broccoli	Potatoes
Brussels sprouts	Sweet potatoes
Guava	Spinach
Mangos	Asparagus
Papayas	Turnip greens

Breads and Cereals

Serve whole grain or restored breads and cereals, and other baked foods made with enriched or whole grain flour. Use four servings daily.

If cereals are not chosen, have an extra serving of any of the foods that are listed here:

Bread	Cornmeal
Rolls	Crackers
Biscuits	Grits
Muffins	Rolled oats
Pancakes	Bulgar
Waffles	Rice
Wheat cereal	Macaroni
Corn cereal	Spaghetti
Oat cereal	Noodles

Daily Food Guide

By the time your baby is eating three meals a day he has probably been exposed to a wide variety of foods. Milk is still the mainstay of the diet, but he will also be drinking orange and other juices. Be sure your baby gets an adequate supply of protein, fresh fruits and vegetables, and whole-grain breads and cereals.

Beginning around the ninth month, and up through the first year, the following amounts of food are recommended each day:

Milk	As needed
Cereal or bread	in moderation
Fruits and Juices	3 servings
Vegetables and Juices	2 servings
Protein Foods	2 servings

Some sample menus are given to provide you with ideas for planning balanced meals. The foods are adequate in all nutrients if consumed in the amounts recommended. As baby gets older and hungrier you may add more of these or other nourishing foods he likes.

Use the menus as references for planning meals. For additional information check the diet sheet provided by your doctor. Starting times and starting foods will vary according to each baby's need.

4-6 Months

(Or when your baby is ready to start) Bananas, avocado, papaya, applesauce or other soft fruits once a day.

6 Months

Cereal in moderation
Fruits twice a day
Vegetables once or twice a day
Meat or egg yolk on doctor's advice

6-8 Months

Egg on doctor's advice
Cereal in moderation
Fruits and juices twice a day
Meat, poultry or fish once or twice a day
Vegetables once or twice a day
Finger foods as needed
Milk and yogurt

9-12 Months

At this age baby should be accustomed to a wide variety of foods. He's probably eating diced meat, hunks of cheese and other nutritious finger foods. A more detailed menu may be helpful now:

Breakfast

Egg on doctor's advice
Cream of Wheat or
    Whole-wheat toast
Orange Juice
Milk

Lunch

Cottage Cheese
Peas
Applesauce
Milk

Dinner

Meat
Potato or Rice
Avocado
Peaches
Milk

Snacks

Finger fruits
Teething vegetables
Milk and fruit juice
Whole-grain breads
Cheese
Yogurt

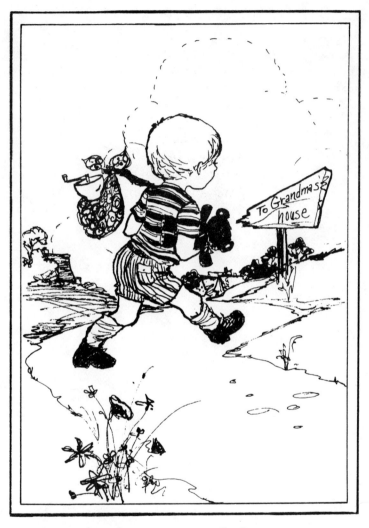

3. How to Use a Baby Food Grinder

Once you start using a baby food grinder you will immediately appreciate its convenience and versatility because you can use it for every meal. It's the most economical and healthful way to prepare your baby's food. With very little effort it quickly transforms semi-solid foods into pureed ones.

A baby food grinder is a very small version of the standard food mill or ricer. It will grind fruits, vegetables and meats directly from the table. Its small size makes it easy to grind small portions of food; it will make as little as a tablespoonful or as much as a small cupful with a few simple turns of the handle. It is so compact you can take it with you when you visit friends, dine out or travel.

Food that is freshly ground has many advantages over food that has been prepared in other ways. Among them: It's a tremendous money and time saver. You can feed fresh fruits in season. The food is usually at the right temperature. You do not have to prepare food in large batches. The baby can eat fresh nourishing food right from the table and you will always know what's in the food you offer him.

Foods pressed through a baby food grinder taste so much better than foods prepared by other methods that there is no comparison. Babies who learn to eat from a grinder, because they have more exposure to a wide variety of foods, will learn to eat almost anything.

Older babies, who have been exposed to mildly seasoned foods, Junior Dinners and Toddler Meals, can enjoy holiday dinners at the table with other children and grownups. It is important to include the baby as part of the family as early as possible because it's fun for him and because it teaches him to develop a taste for new foods.

If given a chance babies are curious and venturesome when it comes to exploring new foods. This is one of the best reasons for feeding your baby from family meals right from the beginning. Foods taste better. It teaches him to sample new foods. And each meal is a new experience that baby will look forward to because it is guaranteed not to taste or feel or chew the same as the previous day's meal.

Once you start using the baby food grinder regularly you will discover that babies enjoy, as well as prefer, freshly ground food over foods prepared in other ways. There is a very good reason for this preference. Baby's appetite, like that of grownups, is stimulated by the pleasant aromas that come from foods that are cooking. Babies like to be offered food that tastes like the food they smell.

As the months go by and baby continues to grow and develop you can make the food chewier, lumpier and more varied. Eventually, as baby's appetite grows, all of his food can be selected from the adult menus you and your family like best. You may also find the family's meals getting better and better nutritionally as you try out for yourself some of the foods that are good for baby. Once you become concerned about balancing the diet for your baby you'll also care more about balancing the diet for the rest of the family.

If you have your baby food grinder handy in the kitchen, or take it wherever you go, the baby can start early to participate in the basic family function of eating together and enjoying mother's cooking. Another nice feature about a baby food grinder is that the skins of peas, hulls of corn and strings from green beans are not mixed in with the food. They stay under the cutting blade. These hard-to-digest particles are easily discarded after the baby is fed the ground portion.

Once you begin to use the grinder regularly you'll find other uses for it too. You can make sandwich spreads and instant milk and fruit drinks for the entire family. The baby food grinder is also helpful for older children or anyone that has an illness requiring pureed foods.

Traveling and Dining Out

Even when you're away from home baby can enjoy his meals right along with everyone else. When traveling or dining out take the baby food grinder along. Take it to other peoples' houses too and let the baby eat a spoonful or two of grownup food. It makes visiting much easier.

Take the baby food grinder to restaurants. You can use it all of the time and let the baby eat his dinner right along with everyone else. Specially prepared foods are unnecessary. They're not too practical either because they're usually not the right temperature by the time everyone is ready to eat.

Traveling and dining out is another way of introducing babies to new tastes. Just think what fun it is to sample "adult" food from your plate. It's bound to make little ones feel more grown-up.

When dining out, babies who are accustomed to eating Junior Dinners and Toddler Meals enjoy fresh crab and shrimp, not to mention steak and chops. If possible, select a dinner from the menu that includes a vegetable and/or rice and baked potato. Avoid international dishes; they're a bit too sophisticated for babies.

Soft Foods First

If your baby is just beginning to eat solids you will need to refer to the first two chapters of this book for additional information. The first foods to be given should always be soft foods, either cereals or fruits that have been pressed through the baby food grinder. You may also grind poached, scrambled or boiled eggs and thin the puree with milk until the desired consistency is reached, if there is no allergy.

As the baby graduates to Junior Dinners and Toddler Meals he should be able to handle any of the foods nicely just as they come out of the grinder. The important thing to remember is don't force tough cuts of meat or other chewy foods through the grinder. *If you can't grind it, don't feed it to the baby.*

If you have started with cereals you are ready to switch to fruit. You can start by pressing a small portion of completely ripe banana through the grinder and mixing it with a little milk. Apricots, apples, peaches, pears and prunes are all popular with babies. A baby food grinder will grind these fruits into smooth textures readily acceptable by the baby.

Cooked apples can be turned into instant applesauce when pressed through the grinder. As soon as baby is able to handle fresh fruits try fresh apples. They are absolutely delicious and need no cooking before pureeing in the baby food grinder. When you start any fruits, thin the pureed mixture with milk. It's not necessary to add sugar to any of the fruits.

Use any fresh or canned fruits you have prepared for the family. If the fruit is packed in syrup rinse it off before grinding. For variety, fruits and vegetables may be ground in any combination that baby may enjoy. When preparing cooked cereal for the family press it through the grinder with a little fruit before serving baby. Also remember that all fruits blend deliciously with cottage cheese.

When you're ready to begin vegetables use soft-cooked ones or combinations of vegetables that you have prepared for the family. For nutrition and flavor use fresh vegetables whenever possible. Frozen vegetables are the best substitute for fresh. They also save on time since washing and cutting are already done. Canned vegetables may also be used. Whenever possible use the liquid, as many nutrients are in it. When preparing the family's meal be sure to set aside a portion for baby before adding salt or fat. Add natural juices to the ground food if necessary.

As the baby adjusts to eating solids you can go to cheese, chicken, fish and meats. Use soft-cooked, steamed, stewed, roasted, or braised meats, poultry or fish. After grinding add pan juices or some other unsalted liquid to thin the food.

As the baby gets used to the different textures you can decrease the amount of liquid that you earlier added to the ground food. Eventually he'll be eating most foods just as they come out of the baby food grinder. He'll have no trouble at all swallowing thicker or coarser mixtures if you gradually reduce the amount of liquid added to the ground food.

Since babies are susceptible to digestive upsets it's important to handle food properly during its preparation. Be certain that your hands are clean and that you work with clean utensils.

A baby food grinder is simply constructed and easy to keep clean. Wash and rinse in hot water after each use.

Combination and Junior Dinners

Grind beef, lamb, veal, chicken, fish or organ meats right from the table. Thin the ground mixture with a little cooking liquid, milk, pan juices or gravy. To make a Meat Pie, top with a dollop of mashed potatoes before offering to baby.

To make a stew, add any combinations of meat, carrots, squash, peas or other cooked greens. For Irish Stew combine ground breast of lamb, cooked potatoes and boiled onions. To make a fish dinner combine rice, fish and hard-cooked eggs. Add a little milk and butter for flavor.

Moisten ground cooked liver with cooking juice or water. Add an equal portion of soft mashed potato. If the food is not warm from the table you may need to heat it in a covered saucepan over low heat on the top of the stove. As the baby is able to tolerate more mixtures of food you can make a complete dinner in a dish by adding carrots or other soft, cooked vegetables that you have pressed through the baby food grinder.

As the baby's tastes become more sophisticated try adding cooked sweet peppers and boiled onions to the liver. Babies will frequently eat liver prepared with braised celery, tomatoes and carrots even though they refuse to eat it in other forms. Other babies may enjoy a mixture of ground liver, beef, cooked oatmeal and tomatoes. Also see Chapter 8, "Liver Dinner," for a good way to introduce iron-rich liver to babies who think they don't like it.

Some babies prefer a combination of ground chicken liver and applesauce. A liver spread can be made by mixing together cottage cheese and green pepper. Spread on triangles of whole wheat bread and serve as finger food.

Kidneys, heart, tongue and other organ meats can be used in place of beef. Combine any of them with other vegetables just as you would in making stew. Only season the stew after the baby's portion is removed from the cooking pot. Or allow an older baby to have any mild seasonings enjoyed by the rest of the family.

When preparing organ meats remove any fat, membranes, gristle or blood vessels before pressing through the baby food grinder. If you cannot grind the organ meats then you should not feed them to the baby.

To make a delicious sandwich spread add a little cooking liquid and softened cream cheese to the ground meat. Vegetables may also be added to the spread. Organ meats may be blended with cream sauce and served on toast once the baby is able to handle finger foods well. For older babies grind a little cooked green pepper and boiled onions and mix it with the cream sauce before blending in the organ meats.

Soups can be made out of any of these Combination Dinners by adding water and milk, broth and milk, and vegetable juices and milk. Or if desired, plain water may be used. When adding vegetables to soup use only those vegetables that have already been introduced into your baby's diet. Use barley, macaroni, noodles and rice sparingly as they are basically filler foods. See Chapter 10 for additional information on making soups.

Try grinding walnuts, raisins and cream cheese for a nutritious sandwich spread. A combination of cottage cheese, pears or apples and raisins and walnuts make a tasty fruit salad.

Some Ways to Thin Baby's Food

A food's own natural juices are usually enough to give baby's meals an agreeable consistency. But sometimes fruit juice, or an addition like applesauce, yogurt or cottage cheese may be needed to enhance the texture of ground meat, poultry or fish. This is particularly true in early infancy when your baby is eating mostly soft-cooked foods.

Whatever the case, your baby will let you know what he likes best. Choose from any of the following:

Fruit Juice

Fresh or canned fruit juice, when mixed with other foods, will help baby's food slip down a little easier. Don't forget to use the liquid from steamed and stewed fruits as it's also high in food value. Fruit liquid can be used to thin fruit or vegetable puree.

Vegetable Juice

To get the full nutritive value from cooked vegetables always use the liquid in the pan in some other way. Add it to soup, meat, or pureed vegetables. Canned vegetable juices may be used for this purpose too.

Meat Broths and Pan Juices

Mix meat broths with vegetables, mashed potatoes, pureed beans and rice. Also use meat broth to moisten ground meat and mixtures of meat, fruit and cottage cheese.

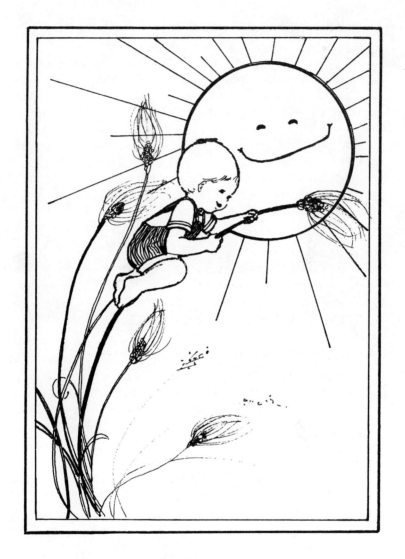

4. Cereals

Cereal is commonly given as baby's first solid food. As it is not meant to be the bulk of the diet, use cereal only in moderation.

There are some babies who do not like cereal at all. If your baby feels this way, report it to your doctor and start with fruit. Babies are usually able to get enough calories from milk and a variety of different solid foods. Sufficient iron is available from a variety of purple fruits, green vegetables, meats and egg yolk. In other words, grains and starches are the things you need to worry about least in your baby's diet. Also note that cereals and breads, when consumed in excess, are one of the primary causes of infantile obesity.

If you give cereal as baby's first solid food, start with rice and oat cereal. After a few months switch over to wheat, corn and barley, and later, the mixed ones, if there is no allergy. Also, check with your doctor before adding egg yolk to the cereal as some babies cannot tolerate egg.

Dried fruits and raisins may be stirred in while cooking, or after cooking, to provide sweetening and added nourishment. Fresh fruits should be pressed through a baby food grinder and blended with the cereal just before serving. For additional information refer to the chapter on Fruits and Juices.

Some babies as they get a little older get bored with cereal and egg dishes for breakfast. When this happens try offering whole-grain breads with cheese, or fruit and cheese spreads. Chapter 11, "Snack Foods," gives ideas for varying the breakfast menu. Also see Chapter 7, "Eggs."

Old-Fashioned Oats

3/4 cup water or milk
1/3 cup old-fashioned oats

Bring liquid to a boil. Sprinkle oats in slowly so the boiling does not stop. Cook 5 minutes longer, stirring occasionally. For a creamier cereal put oats in cold liquid before bringing to a boil. Cover, remove from heat, and let stand until lukewarm. Press the oatmeal through a baby food grinder just before serving.

Rolled Oats and Banana

1/4 cup rolled oats
1/2 cup water or milk
1/3 ripe banana
1/4 cup milk

Combine rolled oats and 1/2 cup of water or milk. Bring to a boil. Simmer for 5 minutes, stirring occasionally. Remove from heat. Cover and let stand for 5 minutes.

Slice banana, and puree in a baby food grinder; add remaining milk, mixing thoroughly. Stir the banana-milk mixture into the cooked cereal.

Cornmeal Mush

1/2 cup water
1/4 cup cornmeal

Bring water to a full boil in the top of a double boiler. Slowly stir in cornmeal. Cook 15 minutes or longer, stirring occasionally.

Cereal Flakes

1/2 cup barley, rice, rye or
wheat cereal flakes
1 cup boiling water

Stir the cereal flakes into a pan containing boiling water. Reduce heat. Cook barley flakes for 5 minutes; rice flakes for 3 to 4 minutes; rye flakes, stirring occasionally, 15 to 20 minutes; and wheat flakes, stirring occasionally, for 6 to 7 minutes. Pureed fruit may be stirred in at serving time.

Cereal a la Mode

cooked Cream of Rice,
Cream of Wheat, or
oatmeal
fruit puree

Puree applesauce, apricots, bananas, peaches, pineapple or prunes in a baby food grinder. Thin with a little milk and spoon on top of the cereal.

It is better to use fresh or freshly cooked fruits without sugar. Canned fruits are all right too, as long as you rinse the syrup off before you puree the fruit in the baby food grinder.

Cream of Wheat Cereal

1 cup water or milk
1 tablespoon Cream of Wheat Cereal

Bring liquid to a boil. Sprinkle the cereal in slowly so that the boiling does not stop. Cook for 15 minutes or until thickened, stirring frequently.

Cream of Rice Cereal

2/3 cup water or milk
1 tablespoon Cream of Rice Cereal

Bring liquid to a boil. Sprinkle the cereal in slowly so that the boiling does not stop. Cook over low heat for 5 minutes, stirring occasionally. Cool.

Fruit Blended Cereals

cooked Cream of Rice,
Cream of Wheat, or
oatmeal
fruit puree

Add pureed raisins, apricots, prunes or some other fruit to cooked cereal. You may blend it in thoroughly or revel it. Or, cook the pureed fruit right along with the cereal.

When making fruit puree in a baby food grinder be careful not to offer any chunks of fruit pulp that remain beneath the cutting blade.

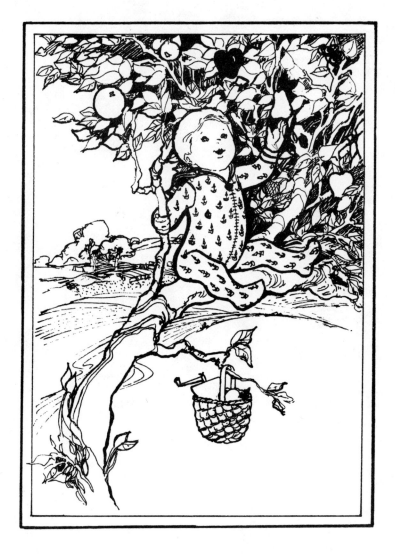

5. Fruits and Juices

Applesauce and raw mashed banana are well liked by babies and for this reason are frequently given as the first solid food in place of cereal.

Increase each fruit gradually as the baby learns to like it. Whenever possible, use fresh fruits without sugar. If it is necessary to peel a fruit, peel it very thinly. If fresh fruits are not available, the next best choice is frozen or canned fruits that have been packed in water.

If your doctor recommends hard or dried fruits, steam the fruit just long enough to soften the fibers. Use only enough water to prevent the fruit from scorching, and cover the pan to prevent the steam from escaping. If you follow these pointers the fruit you cook will have more food value, better color, flavor and texture.

Most babies, over four months of age, are able to tolerate their fruit fresh, including tropical fruits, melons and some berries. The only requirement is that all fresh fruits be thoroughly ripened and soft. If you are using canned fruits packed in syrup rinse off the fruit before grinding. Also be sure to discard any fruit pulp or seeds that stick to the back of the cutting blade.

If you have any doubts about offering your baby strawberries and other berries check with your doctor. This is advisable for two reasons. The seeds in berries can irritate young digestive systems. These foods can also cause allergic reactions in some babies.

Never give your baby whole berries or bits of fruit the size of peas; they can be swallowed the wrong way causing baby to choke. Dried fruits can be pureed, cooked or uncooked. They are good in cereals or spread on finger-sized pieces of whole-grain bread. Fruits which can be given to baby during his first year are:

Hard or Dried Cooked Fruits	Soft, Ripened Fresh Fruits
Apples	Apples
Apricots	Bananas
Peaches	Pears
Pears	Peaches
Plums	Avocados
Prunes	Oranges
Figs	Berries on
Raisins	doctor's advice
Pineapple	Melons
Other dried fruits	Tropical fruits

Fresh Fruit Puree

fresh fruit
use apricots, bananas, pears, peaches,
berries or tropical fruits

Thoroughly wash well-ripened fruit and peel if necessary. Press through a baby food grinder and serve immediately.

Do not give the baby any pieces of fruit pulp that may have adhered to the bottom of the cutting blade.

Cooked Fruit Puree

fresh, frozen or canned fruit
use apples, apricots, peaches,
pears, plums, prunes, pineapple
or dried fruits

Wash and peel fruit if necessary. Steam over low heat with a small amount of water until tender. Do not overcook. Cool and press through the baby food grinder. Serve.

Fruit Juices

**fresh fruit
use oranges, pears, melons,
    pineapple, mangos, papaya or
    any fruit with a high moisture
    content**

Thoroughly wash the fruit and peel if necessary. Cut into small cubes and press through the baby food grinder. Pour into a small cup or glass. Be sure to discard any pieces of fruit pulp that may have collected under the cutting blade.

A little freshly squeezed orange juice may be added to any of the juices that have been prepared this way. Also mix canned fruit juices with fresh fruit puree. Try combining ½ cup orange juice with ¼ cup any other fruit. You may also blend ½ cup apple juice with ¼ cup fruit. Or make some of the following combinations:

Orange-Pineapple	Pineapple-Mango
Orange-Apricot	Orange-Pear
Pineapple-Banana	Orange-Apple
Prune-Orange	Watermelon-Orange
Banana-Orange	Apple-Peach
Apricot-Pear	Apple-Grape
Mango-Pear	Apple-Plum

Fruit juices made in a food grinder will have a consistency similar to unfiltered juices. They will be somewhat thick. In early infancy dilute them with a little water before feeding to baby. Save the more sophisticated fruit blends, drinks and shakes for older babies.

Tomato Juice

**use fresh tomatoes that have been
dipped into hot water and peeled**

Cut a tomato into wedges and press through the
baby food grinder. Press the tomatoes through slowly
so the juice does not splash out. You can prevent this if
you press most of the liquid into the grinder container
before turning the handle to puree the pulp. Discard
the stem end and any pulp that may stick to the cutting
blade.

Tomato juice that has been pureed this way can be
mixed with meat, macaroni or cheese. If you add a
little milk and heat you will have fresh tomato soup.
Any vegetables from the family meal can be mixed
with the tomato juice.

Fruit Slush

**use combinations of fruit, orange
juice or cooked pureed carrots**

Thoroughly ripened melons, berries and tropical
fruits can be combined with a spoonful of banana to
make other fruit slushes. A combination of pineapple
juice and pureed carrots makes another very tasty
slush. Surprisingly, so do equal parts of orange juice
and carrots.

Orange, pineapple, apple or grape juice, or
combinations of these, may be mixed with pureed dry
fruit. A little grapefruit juice can be added to perk up
the flavor. Taste for sweetness as you go along.

Apple Slush

1 small fresh apple
banana puree

Peel the apple and cut into chunks. Press through the baby food grinder. Pour into a cup and add about a tablespoonful of pureed banana. Mix well and feed to baby.

Instant Fruit Butter

raisins, prunes, dates,
figs or dried pineapple
milk

Use any of the above dried fruits or a mixture of dried fruit such as apricots, peaches, pears and pineapple. Dried fruits that are plump and moist can be made into butters without any cooking. And a baby food grinder will puree them quite readily without having to soak or steam the fruit in water, although, if necessary, this can be done.

You may want to start with a spoonful of raisins to see how easily fruit butter can be made. The pureed fruit will be quite thick so thin it with a little milk until the desired consistency is reached.

Mix fruit butter with cottage cheese, pureed carrots or peanut butter and spread on pieces of whole-grain bread. A combination of dried pineapple and cottage cheese makes a delicious spread. Fruit butters may also be spooned onto pieces of celery. Be sure to remove the strings from the celery so baby won't choke on them.

Fruit Combo

**fresh, frozen or canned fruit
use combinations of baby's
favorite fruits**

Babies never outgrow fruits but they may lose interest in certain ones. Should this happen you can continue to please them by mixing several fruits together:

Apples and Apricots	Prunes and Pears
Bananas and Peaches	Mango and Banana
Pineapple and Pears	Peaches and Pears
Plums and Applesauce	Pineapple and Bananas
Bananas and Pineapple	Papaya and Banana
Apricots and Peaches	Plums and Peaches
Apples and Prunes	Mango and Orange

Fruit Puree with Other Foods

**fruit puree
yogurt, cottage cheese,
meat or other baby foods**

Using fruit puree as a base, mix in one or more baby foods.

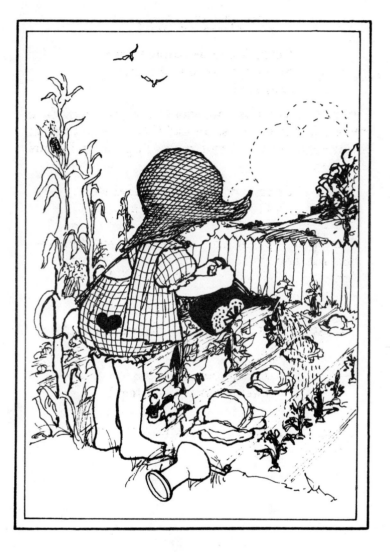

6. Vegetables

After the baby has gotten used to cereal and fruit, pureed vegetables can be added to the diet. Carrots, peas, beets, spinach, squash, sweet potatoes, asparagus, beans and potatoes are recommended first because they are the easiest to digest.

Strong-tasting vegetables such as broccoli, cauliflower, brussels sprouts, cabbage and turnips may also be given. If baby can tolerate these vegetables there is no limit to the different kinds he may have. Remember, a little applesauce or some other fruit can be mixed with strong-tasting vegetables to enhance their flavor.

Don't cook vegetables too long as you will destroy both food value and taste. Excessive cooking will turn the vegetable to mush and cause it to lose its color. Vegetables should be cut in small pieces and simmered in just enough water to prevent scorching. To shorten cooking time have the water boiling before the vegetables are added. Vegetables prepared this way are high in food value and have good color, flavor and texture.

You may also use fresh or fresh-frozen vegetables and canned ones without salt. Use any unseasoned baked or steamed vegetables you may have prepared for the family meal. This is the simplest way to get baby's vegetables. All you have to do is press them through the baby food grinder.

For a nutritious sandwich spread mix pureed carrots with equal amounts of peanut butter.

Beans are good for your baby too because they are another source of iron in the diet. Cook the beans the usual way. If you soak them be sure to use the same water in which the beans were soaked for cooking so that you don't lose the minerals and vitamins that come out of the beans into the soaking water.

There are several other things to remember when preparing beans for the baby. Do not add soda to the water. Do not put bacon, fat, salt or chili in the beans.

When the beans are cooked press them through the baby food grinder. Before offering beans to baby throw away the skin of the beans that collect under the cutting blade. Thin with milk or water.

First Vegetables	*Second Vegetables*
Asparagus	Cabbage
Beets	Turnips
Carrots	Broccoli
Corn	Cauliflower
Green beans	Brussels sprouts
Peas	Kohlrabi
Squash	Lentils
Sweet Potatoes	Dried peas
Spinach	Dried beans

Steamed Vegetables

1 cup fresh vegetables, diced
use carrots, asparagus, squash,
beets, beans, or peas
1/4 cup water

Wash vegetables and peel only if necessary. Steam over low heat until tender. Keep saucepan tightly covered adding additional liquid if necessary. Do not overcook. Cool and press through a baby food grinder. Discard any fibers that may stick to the bottom of the cutting blade.

If any liquid is left in the pan it may be used to thin the vegetable puree. Add the liquid slowly until the right consistency is reached.

Creamed Vegetables

**1 cup fresh vegetables, shredded
carrots, green beans, asparagus,
squash, spinach or potatoes
1/3 cup milk**

Add washed shredded vegetables to the milk. Steam over low heat until done. Keep saucepan tightly covered adding more milk if necessary. Cool and press through the baby food grinder. If necessary, thin with additional milk.

The sweet mild flavor of carrots and peas is greatly enhanced when steamed quickly in a small amount of milk.

Vegetables au Gratin

**pureed vegetables or potatoes
cottage cheese or another mild
    cheese that has been shredded
milk**

Put a serving of pureed vegetables into a small dish. Press about a tablespoonful of cottage cheese through the baby food grinder. Thin with a little milk, warm and pour over the vegetables.

If using some other mild cheese melt it in a little milk before pouring it over the vegetable.

If meats have already been introduced to baby they can be added to Vegetables au Gratin. You may use ground beef, veal, poultry, lamb or liver. Sweet vegetables, like yams, squash, carrots, peas and corn make tasty dinners when mixed with ground meats. To make Toddler Meals combine diced vegetables with the meat.

Mashed Potato Special

potato
hot milk
pureed vegetables

Puree the potatoes and add hot milk. Beat until fluffy. Heat the vegetable and serve in the center of a mound of pureed potatoes.

To make a Toddler Meal, use diced vegetables instead of pureed ones. Diced meat or cheese can also be used in place of vegetables.

Sweet Potato with Avocado

sweet potato
avocado

Combine pureed sweet potato and avocado. Steamed squash or carrots may be used in place of the sweet potato.

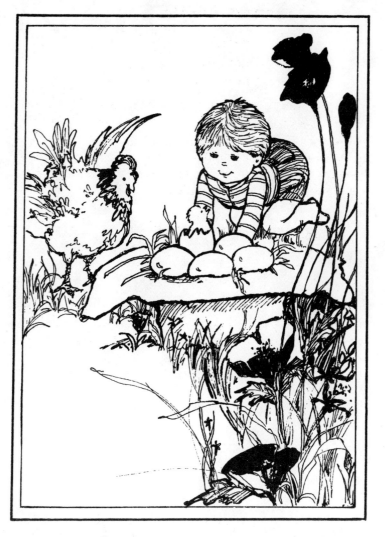

7. Eggs

When your doctor first suggests eggs as part of your baby's diet he may tell you to offer the yolk raw, or the egg cooked. Always start with the yolk, as it's the white that usually causes an allergic reaction.

Never overcook eggs. The white gets tough and the yolk mealy. Moisture is important so never offer a baby a dry yolk. Use fresh eggs and cook them carefully if you expect baby to eat them.

Egg yolk can be mixed with cereal, fruit, vegetables or meat. You may scramble them with milk or a little cottage cheese. Whether eggs are served plain or more elegantly, keep them moist. As baby gets older make egg salad sandwiches and omelets. Eggs can be added to creamed soup and other hot dishes. Don't forget to use the baby food grinder to make egg salad for the entire family.

When the baby is able to handle Toddler Meals you may want to offer him something different for breakfast. Babies like a change now and then. Here are several ways to get variety — and maybe surprises — into breakfast.

For a different flavor treat, sprinkle grated cheese over eggs to be baked, or combine with scrambled eggs. Eggs can be scrambled with tomato puree. Potatoes and eggs can also be scrambled together. Cheese and chopped meat may be given for breakfast. Serve these as alternates for eggs.

Split rolls, muffins or cornbread and spread with scrambled eggs or any of the fillings in Chapter 11. Pureed meat, grated cheese and egg also go well on toast. Try adding tomato juice to the egg and milk mixture when making French Toast. Some Toddlers enjoy their French Toast spread with just a little bit of peanut butter.

Scrambled Egg

1 egg, beaten
1 tablespoon milk
butter, unsalted

Combine egg with milk and beat thoroughly. Melt butter in a small saucepan and cook egg slowly over low heat, stirring occasionally until done.

Cottage cheese, other mild cheeses and chopped vegetables can be added to eggs as baby gets older.

Cereal and Egg

2/3 cup milk
1 tablespoon Cream of Rice Cereal
1 egg, beaten

Heat milk in a saucepan. Slowly stir in Cream of Rice, stirring for 1 minute. Simmer gently 4 minutes longer.

Dilute the egg with a small amount of hot cereal and stir it into the remaining hot cereal. Cook for 1 more minute, remove from heat and cool.

Fruit puree can be blended with cereal and egg to make a tasty breakfast. Just before serving press the cereal and fruit through a baby food grinder.

Eggs Marvelous

scrambled egg
fruit puree

Stir baby's favorite fruit into scrambled egg. Garnish with a dollop of yogurt.

French Toast

1 egg, beaten
2 tablespoons milk
whole-grain bread
butter, unsalted
fruit topping

Beat egg and milk together. Soak bread in mixture until thoroughly saturated. Saute in butter over moderate heat until lightly browned.

Press baby's favorite fruit through a baby food grinder and spread over the French toast. Cut into strips and serve as finger food.

Spread French Toast with cottage cheese and applesauce. Or top with fresh strawberries and Strawberry Fruit-Blended Yogurt. French Toast with peaches and Peach Yogurt makes an elegant toddler dessert.

Toddler Omelet

1 egg
1 tablespoon milk
1 1/2 teaspoons butter, unsalted
1/4 cup any pureed vegetable

Beat egg slightly. Add milk. Melt butter over low heat in a frying pan. Pour egg mixture into pan. Cook slowly over low heat, carefully lifting sides with a spatula to let uncooked part run underneath. When done, turn onto serving plate. Heat vegetable and spread on top of cooked egg. Fold in half.

Pureed fruit, meat or shredded cheese may be used in place of vegetables. The fruit, vegetables and meat may be diced if the toddler can handle it.

Stuffed Eggs

1 egg, hard-cooked
1 1/2 tablespoons vegetable puree
1 teaspoon melted butter, unsalted

Cut egg in half lengthwise. Remove yolk and put white aside. Puree the yolk in a baby food grinder. Add vegetable and melted butter. Blend well. Refill white with mixture.

You may also use 2 1/2 to 3 1/2 tablespoons pureed beef, chicken, veal, lamb or liver in place of vegetables. If needed, use some milk to thin the meat and egg yolk mixture.

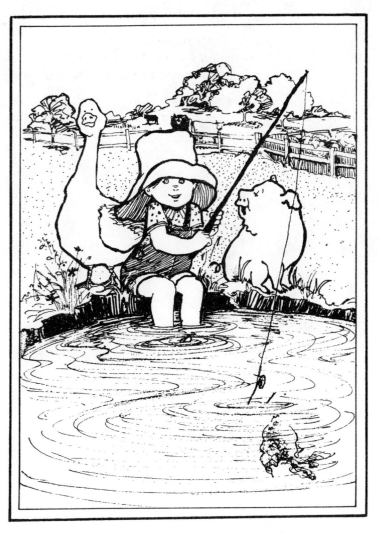

8. Meat, Poultry and Fish

Before adding meat to baby's diet it is best to check with your doctor. He may ask you to wait six months or longer before introducing meat.

Meat, chicken and turkey or any bland-flavored fish that you have cooked for your family can be used to make baby-sized dinners. There is no need to go through any special effort to prepare these foods either, as long as there's a baby food grinder nearby. Do keep in mind, however, to set aside a portion for baby before adding salt and other seasonings for the rest of the family.

When preparing meat for the rest of the family cook it at a low temperature; this helps to preserve its food value. Meat that is overcooked or cooked at too high a temperature also loses its flavor.

If you have prepared a roast for the rest of the family set aside a softly-cooked lean portion. When the baby is ready to eat cut the meat into small pieces and press it through the food grinder. Just add cooked vegetables, a little pan juices, milk or some other liquid to make it palatable for baby.

Since meat and poultry have a grainy texture when pureed, it is necessary to combine them with some other food so they will slip down easily. Cream of Rice Cereal that has been set aside from breakfast, can be mixed with pureed meats to give a smoother consistency. Some very tasty dinners can be made by combining fruits with the meat puree.

Pureed poultry, however, is so bland-tasting that Cream of Rice Cereal does not improve its flavor. It is best to mix poultry with an equal amount of vegetables or some fruit. Fish is better when mixed with a pureed vegetable or white sauce. Always use only the blandest-flavored fish as this tastes best to babies.

Never give processed, cured, smoked or ready-to-serve luncheon meats to babies. These foods are all highly seasoned and contain far too many preservatives — good reasons why they should not be given to babies.

Use your baby food grinder to puree meat, poultry or fish with fruits, vegetables, cottage cheese, eggs and cereals. Many flavorful combinations can be made. The following guide will get you started.

Combination Dinners

Beef and Bananas
Beef and Cereal
Veal and Applesauce
Lamb and Carrots
Chicken and Peas
Meat and Vegetables
Meat and Sweet Potato
Fish, White Sauce
  and Noodles
Liver and Carrots
Liver, Noodles and
  White Sauce

Turkey and Carrots
Meat and Potatoes
Fish, Peas and
  Cottage Cheese
Meat, Vegetable, and
  Egg Yolk
Meat and Fruit
Turkey and Peas
Meat and Noodles
Poultry, Cottage Cheese
  and Noodles

Junior Dinners

Junior Dinners are made from the soft-cooked foods you have been feeding baby all along. The only difference is that they have a coarser texture. They are not too soft and not too firm. Their main purpose is to help accustom baby to coarser foods and encourage him to eat more of them.

Some of these foods, especially cereals, fruits and eggs, will remain favorites for several years or longer, while interest in other foods may diminish. That is the time for making them more "grown-up." To renew interest in these foods, simply add any mild seasoning, a little salt, a little butter and other mild-flavored condiments.

The following pages present various food combinations that will help you plan meals that are nutritious and tasteful. A large variety of food combinations is suggested because it has been shown that early exposure to many foods develops a wider acceptance of foods in later life. The only thing you need to remember is to introduce the new flavors and textures gradually, just as you did with the soft-cooked foods during early infancy.

The food combinations suggested here are meant to taste like "grown-up" foods because babies react favorably to this approach. The foods suggested are suitable for the entire family, with the slight addition of salt and seasonings. Including these suggestions in family meals is an excellent way to help make little folks part of the family. Babies are social beings and enjoy sharing their Junior Dinners and Toddler Meals with other family members.

Junior
Fruit with Vegetables

Combine fruit and vegetables in equal amounts. Try yellow squash, peas, beans, or any favorite vegetable, mixed with apples, pears or tomatoes.

Junior
Turkey Rice Dinner

Mix together equal amounts of turkey and rice. Tomato puree and carrots will add flavor. Thin with milk until the desired consistency is reached.

Junior
Macaroni and Cheese

Prepare macaroni and cheese for the entire family and puree a portion for baby. Stir in a little milk.

Junior
Mixed Vegetables

Blend together two or more vegetables that your baby likes. Add some pureed meat if desired.

Junior
Split Peas with Sweet Potato

Make Split Pea Soup for the rest of the family and puree several spoonfuls with a few bite-sized pieces of sweet potato.

Junior
Beef and Egg Noodles

Take beef from the family meal and mix it with an equal amount of egg noodles. Thin with milk as needed.

Junior
Vegetables and Liver

Combine two parts of your baby's favorite vegetable with one part of pureed liver and a little cooked onion.

Junior
Chicken Noodle Dinner

Blend together equal parts of chicken, noodles and carrots. Tomato puree may be added for flavor.

Junior
Chicken with Vegetables

Puree equal parts of chicken, potatoes and carrots and mix together.

Junior
Turkey with Vegetables

Combine equal parts of turkey, potatoes and carrots and add just enough tomato puree to flavor.

Junior
Veal with Vegetables

Mix together equal amounts of veal and potatoes. Stir in a spoonful of peas and carrots and add tomato puree to perk up the flavor.

Junior
Beef with Vegetables

Stir together equal amounts of pureed beef and potatoes. Add a spoonful of carrots and peas and a little tomato puree. Mix well.

Toddler Meals

Toddler Meals are composed of mashed or chopped foods, which may or may not include some pureed or ground food.

Prepare fruits, vegetables and meats as usual by pressing them through the food grinder, but add some larger pieces to the mixture. When combining foods of different textures for the first time you will want to use more of the ground food and perhaps reduce the size of the chopped pieces.

When changing over to mashed or chopped foods do it gradually so it won't upset baby's digestion. As your baby grows older, your doctor will tell you what foods your baby needs, when to start them, and how much to give.

During the times the baby is growing slower, he may be less hungry. He may be more choosy and refuse certain foods. Don't worry or force him to eat. Keep on offering different foods. In time, he will likely take the ones he is turning down now.

Toddler
Green Beans, Potatoes and Egg Casserole

Remove any strings from the green beans and cut into small pieces. Add to pureed potatoes and finely chopped egg.

Toddler
Vegetable and Turkey Casserole

Take any two vegetables your baby likes, puree one, and dice the other. Mix this with chopped turkey.

Toddler
Bite-Size Beef Stew

Cut carrots, beef, and potatoes into bite-sized pieces. Mix with pan juices or beef broth.

Toddler
Creamed Potatoes and Peas

Combine creamed potatoes you have fixed for the rest of the family with green peas. If creamed potatoes are not available use plain or mashed potatoes. Thin the mixture with milk. Use one part of potatoes with two parts of peas.

Toddler
Beef Lasagna

Mix ground beef, cut up noodles, cottage cheese and tomato puree together.

Chicken Stew

**use chicken or turkey that has
been prepared for the rest
of the family
milk
carrots or peas
mashed potatoes**

Puree the chicken or turkey in a baby food grinder. Add a little milk to moisten thoroughly. Blend the chicken with carrots or peas and fold into mashed potatoes.

Fish Pie

**use any steamed or baked fish that
the family has for dinner
milk
pureed vegetables or potatoes
shredded cheese**

Press the fish through a baby food grinder and add a little milk to moisten. Top with pureed vegetables or potatoes and garnish with a bit of cheese. Let the Fish Pie warm through for a few minutes until the cheese has melted.

Use only bland-flavored fish; otherwise baby may reject what's offered. A little Cream of Rice cereal may be added to fish to make it more palatable.

Meat Pie

**use pieces of beef, veal, lamb
or organ meats from the
family's dinner
mashed potatoes
butter, unsalted**

Press the meat or organ meats through a baby food grinder. Add a little cooking liquid or gravy to enhance the consistency. Top with whipped mashed potatoes to which you have added a tiny bit of butter.

Liver Dinner

**liver
pieces of cooked onion
butter, unsalted
milk
cooked noodles**

Grind liver and onion together and mix with a dab of butter. Thin with a little milk and blend with noodles that have been pressed through a baby food grinder.

A piece of tomato can be ground with the liver if you like. Also note that some babies prefer their liver mixed with a little applesauce.

Any of these variations are popular, even with babies who think they don't like liver. Left-over liver may be ground and blended with seasonings and cream cheese and served (as a spread on crackers or celery sticks), garnished with egg. Don't forget, you can grind eggs in a baby food grinder.

Goulash

beef cooked in onions
fresh tomato
light cream or milk
cooked noodles or rice

After you have ground the beef and tomato in a baby food grinder blend it with a little cream. Combine the meat mixture with noodles that have been pressed through the grinder. If necessary, add a little more liquid until the right consistency is reached. Cooked rice may be used in place of noodles.

Noodles Stroganoff

beef chunks or lean ground
beef cooked in onion
cooked noodles
light cream or milk

Grind beef and cooked noodles in a baby food grinder. Thin to the right consistency with a little cream.

Cheese Burger

lean ground beef or veal
cottage cheese

Mix two parts ground beef or veal with one part cottage cheese. Form mixture into a patty. Cook until done. For baby: Puree in a baby food grinder. For toddlers: Offer the patty as finger food. You may also add beaten eggs, oatmeal or wheat germ.

Meat Balls

ground meat
mashed potatoes, rice,
oatmeal, or any
other cooked cereal

Combine two parts ground meat with one part potato, rice, oatmeal or cereal. Form the mixture into tiny meat balls. Cook until done. For small babies: Puree the meat balls in a baby food grinder. For toddlers: Offer the meat balls as finger foods.

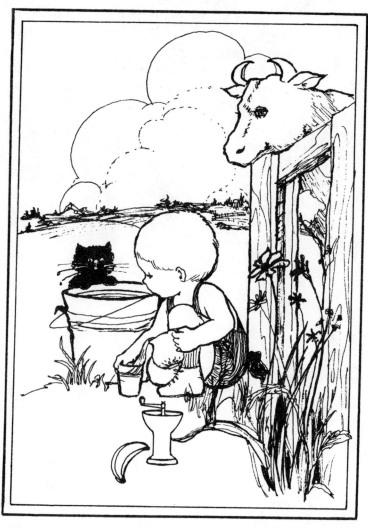

9. Milk Drinks and Dairy Foods

Milk is a basic food which provides babies with a part of the protein needed for growth. Use it in preparing soups, custards, puddings, junkets and cereals. As baby gets older milk can be used in sauces, main dishes and other foods.

When cooking with milk and dairy foods never allow them to boil. Improperly heated milk scorches easily and also causes an off-flavor. Cheese that has been boiled gets stringy and rubbery. Cream sauces need constant stirring while cooking. A double boiler works best for cooking milk mixtures that are thickened. When using dry milk be sure to dissolve it in water before mixing it with other ingredients. Dry milk that hasn't been thoroughly dissolved becomes gummy or chalky.

Cottage cheese, cream cheese and yogurt are all popular and well-tolerated by most babies. Fresh fruit puree and cottage cheese make a nutritious lunch or dessert. Cream cheese can be combined with fruit butters to make a tasty spread on strips of whole-grain bread. See Chapter 11, "Snack Foods."

Most one-year-olds are fond of bite-size cubes of cheese they can pick up with their fingers. They love to chew on it. Other babies prefer their cheese shredded on a cracker.

When fixing Toddler Meals add natural grated cheese to cream sauce. Or grate and use cheese as a topping for vegetables, rice, fish and macaroni dishes. Don't forget toasted cheese sandwiches make good finger foods and add crunch to the diet.

For baby's first dessert mix yogurt with fruit. Milk and pureed fruit can also be combined with canned fruit juices and used as a dessert drink. Use the following guide to prepare tasty milk and fruit drinks.

Milk and Fruit Shakes

Apricot   Fruit and Peanut Butter
Strawberry   Apricot-Pear
Prune   Pineapple-Berry
Cantaloupe   Pineapple-Banana
Tropical Fruit   Peanut Butter-Date
Dried Fruit   Strawberry-Banana
Banana and Peanut Butter   Fruit and Egg

Orange Velvet

1 cup milk
1/4 cup pureed carrots
1 tablespoon orange juice
banana

Thoroughly mix milk and carrots that have been pressed through a baby food grinder. Stir in orange juice and just enough pureed banana to sweeten the drink. Wait until the foam disappears before giving to baby.

Golden Sipper

apricots
carrots
milk

Combine two parts pureed apricots with one part pureed carrots. Add milk until the right consistency is reached.

If you shake the ingredients in a jar with a tight-fitting cover, shake only until thoroughly mixed but not foamy.

Fresh Fruit Shakes

**use bananas, pineapple, cantaloupe,
apricots, strawberries or any
tropical fruits
milk**

When making Fresh Fruit Shakes always use well-ripened fruit. Press the fruit through a baby food grinder and pour into a small cup. Add a little milk and blend thoroughly. Start with equal parts of milk and pureed fruit. Additional milk may be added to thin the mixture. Wait until the foam or bubbles disappear before giving to baby.

Cooked Fruit Puree may also be used in milk shakes. See Chapter 5 for additional information. Milk and banana mixed with a little peanut butter makes another very good shake.

Dried Fruit Shakes

**use any fruit butter
peanut butter
milk**

Prepare fruit butter according to instructions in Chapter 5. Mix equal amounts of fruit butter and peanut butter to form a paste. Gradually add milk and stir until thoroughly blended.

If fruit butters are not used prepare dried fruits according to package directions. Use only a small amount of water to cook dried fruit, just enough to soften the fruit without scorching. Keep what cooking liquids remain in the pan. They can be added to baby's drinks and used to thin fruit puree and other foods.

Eggnog

1 cup milk
1 egg yolk, beaten
banana

Heat milk over low heat. Add beaten egg in a slow stream to hot milk while beating constantly. Use a wire whisk or hand beater. As soon as all the egg has been added remove from heat, cool and chill. Blend in 1/4 cup of banana that has been pressed through a baby food grinder.

Carrot Egg Nog is equally delicious. Substitute 1/4 cup cooked pureed carrots for the banana. Or, add a little banana along with the carrots.

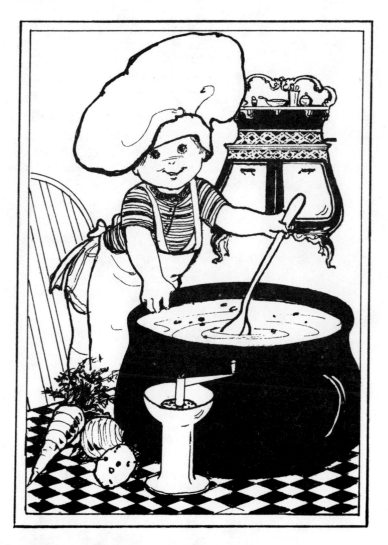

10. Soups

Soups should not be given to baby until he is accustomed to eating a wide variety of mixed foods. The reason for this is to avoid a possible allergic reaction. Just what soups baby will tolerate and at what age are highly individual matters that mother and doctor should decide.

If soups are simple and not too rich or highly seasoned they should be suitable for babies. What baby eats also depends on his digestion, how he has handled various foods in the past, and which ones he dislikes.

Soups that consist of a large amount of filler, such as cereal, rice, barley and noodles, since they contain primarily starch, should not be given to babies. Avoid these fillers when making soups; they're not as nutritious as other foods. Whenever possible rely on broths and stocks to which you have added vegetables and meats.

Once cooked, stocks should be skimmed before using to prepare baby foods. To do this, place the liquid in the refrigerator until cold. When the fat rises to the top remove it with a slotted spoon.

Some mothers like to freeze stocks in ice cube trays. When frozen the cubes are then wrapped in plastic bags, three or four cubes to a bag. They come in very handy to make one baby serving at a time. Also use broths and stocks to flavor baby's vegetables.

Pureed vegetables, meat, fish, poultry and peanut butter can be combined in soups in many different ways to get enough variety to please even the fussiest eater. You can always vary the ingredients to suit your baby's taste. If the soup is too thick to handle, more milk or vegetable juice can be added.

Cream Sauce for Soups

1 cup milk
1 tablespoon Cream of Rice Cereal
1 teaspoon butter, unsalted

Scald milk but do not boil. Slowly stir in cereal and cook for 1 minute, stirring constantly. Remove from heat and let stand for 5 minutes.

For individual servings add 2 tablespoons of pureed vegetables, poultry or meat to 1/4 cup of Cream Sauce. Thin with additional milk if necessary. This basic sauce can be stored in the refrigerator for several days and used as needed.

Vegetable Soup

1 cup Cream Sauce
1/2 cup pureed carrots, peas,
spinach, green beans, lima
beans, corn, garbanzos, lentils
or other beans

Mix Cream Sauce and any of the above vegetables together. Or, combine 2 or more vegetables if you like. Broth or vegetable liquid may be used in place of the Cream Sauce.

Tomato Soup

1 ripe tomato
milk

Peel skin off tomato, cut in cubes and press through a baby food grinder. Add milk and heat.

Meat Soup

1 cup Cream Sauce
1/2 cup pureed lamb, veal or beef

Blend together Cream Sauce and meat that has been pressed through a baby food grinder.

Cheese Soup

1 cup Cream Sauce
1/2 cup chicken broth
1/2 cup shredded cheese

Combine Cream Sauce, broth and any mild-flavored shredded cheese. Heat until cheese melts. Pureed vegetables, fish, poultry or meat may be added to this Cheese Soup. Just wait until serving time before you press additional ingredients through the baby food grinder.

Peanut Butter Soup

1/4 cup cooked potatoes
1/4 cup smooth peanut butter
1/3 cup milk
1 cup Cream Sauce

Press cooked potatoes through a baby food grinder and set aside. Mix peanut butter and milk until thoroughly blended, adding milk a little at a time. Stir in Cream Sauce and potatoes.

Make Tomato-Peanut Butter Soup by blending together milk, pureed tomatoes and a tiny spoonful of peanut butter.

Fruit Soup

apricots
peaches
pears
milk

Prepare fruits according to directions in Chapter 5. Blend equal parts of fruit and milk, heat until warm and serve.

This soup is also good served cold, especially when baby is teething. Buttermilk may be used in place of the milk.

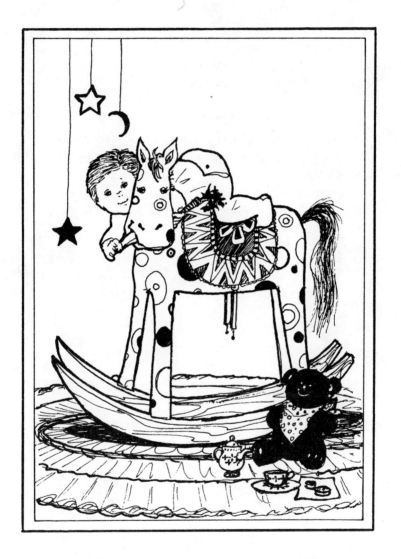

11. Snack Foods

Many good foods are available for between-meal snacks. Whether you choose to offer them or not will depend on baby's appetite. Some babies need mid-morning and mid-afternoon snacks; others do not. It's best not to encourage snacks if baby does not seem to need them.

For those who need extra feedings it's wise to choose wholesome nourishing foods. What you serve him depends on his age and whether he is accustomed to eating coarser foods. Whole-grain bread, fruit, fruit juice, carrot and celery sticks and the milk drinks in Chapter 9 all make nourishing snacks.

Try offering whole-grain breads with cheese, or fruit and cheese spreads. Some babies prefer their bread toasted because it's crunchy and chewy. Be sure to cut it into finger-sized pieces so that it can be handled easily.

Don't be surprised if baby eats only the spread at first. This is because the spread is soft and moist. It's exactly what he's been used to all along. Since he's inclined to eat only the spread make it a nutritious one, mildly flavored and simply prepared, without seasonings.

You can create all kinds of exciting combinations with pureed fruits, meats, fish, vegetables, dried fruits and peanut butter. All you need is a binder of cream, milk, cottage cheese or cream cheese. The following suggestions will get you started.

Cheese and Fruit

Grind a mild natural cheese and fruit in the baby food grinder. Blend together and thin with milk.

Toasted Cheese

Sprinkle shreds of mild-flavored cheese on whole-grain bread. Broil until the cheese starts to bubble. Cool and cut into finger-size pieces before serving.

Chicken and Cream Cheese

Press dark chicken meat through a baby food grinder and blend with a little softened cream cheese. Thin with milk or cream.

Fruit Butter and Cream Cheese

Prepare fruit butter according to the directions in Chapter 5. Blend with an equal amount of softened cream cheese. Thin with milk or cream.

Egg Salad

A baby food grinder makes egg salad to perfection. After you have pureed a hard-cooked egg bind it with cream and a little softened cream cheese.

Raisins and Peanut Butter

Combine an equal amount of pureed raisin and peanut butter. Dates, pineapple, prunes, apricots, carrots and pureed vegetables may also be blended with peanut butter to make sandwich spreads and fillings.

Pineapple and Cream Cheese

Puree pineapple in a baby food grinder and blend with softened cream cheese. Prunes may be used in place of pineapple.

Tutti Frutti Cheese

1/4 cup cottage cheese
1/4 cup fresh fruit puree
2 tablespoons orange or apple juice

Puree the cottage cheese in a baby food grinder. Combine with fruit puree and juice. Less juice may be added if desired. Pour into a cup and serve with a spoon.

Toddlers may prefer their Tutti Frutti Cheese with diced fruit. Serve chilled or at room temperature.

Carrot-Chicken Filling

1/2 cup pureed chicken
2 tablespoons carrot puree
2 tablespoons finely chopped celery
1 tablespoon softened cream cheese

Combine ingredients. Blend well and chill. Pureed beef, veal or pork may be used in place of chicken.

Some toddlers enjoy shredded raw carrot in this filling. About 1 1/2 teaspoons salad dressing may be used in place of the cream cheese.

Peanut Butter-Fruit Special

1/4 cup cottage cheese
2 tablespoons peanut butter
1/4 cup any pureed fruit

Put cottage cheese through a baby food grinder. Blend thoroughly with the peanut butter and pureed fruit. Spread on toast squares or wheat crackers.

Toddlers may find diced fruit more pleasing than pureed fruit.

Banana Sandwiches

whole wheat bread
peanut butter
bananas

Spread whole wheat bread with peanut butter and top with thin slices of banana. Cut into quarters and offer as finger food.

Fruit puree may be used in place of the peanut butter.

Toddler Tidbits

fresh fruit
natural cheese
meat
raisins

Cut fruit, cheese and meat into small cubes and arrange on a plate. Add a few raisins to spark interest and serve as toddler snacks.

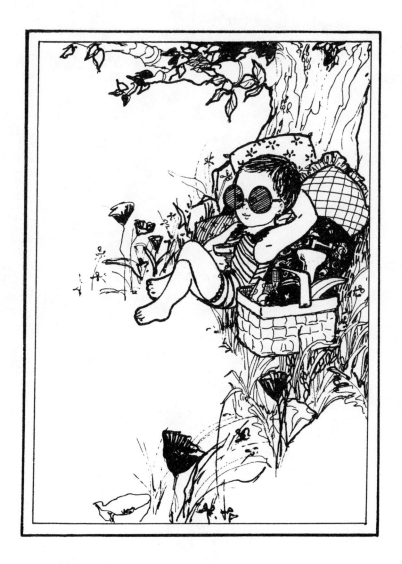

12. Desserts

Serve fruits for baby's dessert. Next to fruits, puddings, junkets and custards are preferred. Cakes, pies, cookies and other concentrated sweets should never be given to babies. Desserts are extras. They are not meant to be offered in place of other nourishing foods.

Healthful desserts can be made by combining equal amounts of plain yogurt and pureed fruit. Cottage cheese and fruit or rice and pureed fruit also make quick nourishing desserts.

Always keep desserts for babies simple and do not offer them between meals as they are likely to dull appetites. The important thing to remember is to use desserts in moderation and select only those with a low sugar content. Carefully chosen desserts can be wholesome.

Sweet potatoes and apples and rice mixed with peaches, apricots, pears or pineapple make nutritious fruit puddings. Pureed apples, apricots, pears and pineapple are quite pleasing when spooned over diced or mashed bananas. Custards and other puddings can be used as a topping on crumbled graham crackers, rusks or zwieback. Don't overlook combining baby's favorite fruit with rice cereal or custard.

Frozen fruit juice and yogurt are another pleasing way to satisfy the "sweet tooth." Blend together two parts yogurt and one part undiluted frozen fruit juice concentrate and freeze.

Toddlers enjoy diced fruit with a soft creamy topping like yogurt or pudding. Peach Fruit-Blended Yogurt makes a marvelous dessert when folded into thickened peach juice gelatin. Refrigerate until set. Some mothers may want to whip the gelatin until fluffy before blending in the yogurt. Try other flavors of yogurt, fruit juice and gelatin for fun.

Junior Desserts

Junior
Hawaiian Delight

Puree any tropical fruits in season and blend with a little pudding or mashed banana.

Junior
Bananas with Pineapple

Combine equal amounts of pureed banana and pineapple. Apples, apricots and pears are quite pleasing too when mixed with banana.

Junior
Applesauce and Apricots

Mix together equal amounts of cooked apples and apricots.

Junior
Dutch Apple Dessert

Blend together cooked apples and pudding. A tiny amount of cinnamon may be added for flavor.

Junior
Peach Melba

Peaches that have been pressed through a baby food grinder can be mixed with pudding. For a Toddler Dessert, spoon the Peach Melba over crumbled zwieback.

Junior
Blueberry Buckle

Press blueberries through a baby food grinder and discard any pulp. Mix with pudding.

First-Tooth Spoon Cooler

1/2 papaya, peeled and seeded
1 small ripe banana
1 ripe peach, peeled
1/2 cup plain yogurt
1/2 cup milk

Peel fruit and cut into cubes. Press prepared fruit through a baby food grinder and blend thoroughly with yogurt and milk. Pour into an ice cube tray and freeze until slushy. This Spoon Cooler tastes best when it's slushy. If frozen solid, thaw to a slushy stage before offering to baby.

Cold fruit mixtures are very refreshing to baby's gums when he is teething. Other sugarless fruit mixtures that have been blended with plain yogurt or yogurt and milk can be used to soothe baby's gums too.

Tasty Fruit Pudding

2/3 cup milk
1 tablespoon Cream of Rice Cereal
2 egg yolks, beaten
pureed banana, pears, peaches, applesauce or prunes

Scald milk in a double boiler. Slowly stir in Cream of Rice and continue to cook for 1 minute, stirring constantly. Cover and simmer gently 4 minutes longer. Stir a little of the hot mixture into the egg yolk and then, stirring constantly, add the yolk to the hot mixture. Continue cooking for 1 more minute. Remove from heat and cool.

Press baby's favorite fruit through a baby food grinder just before serving.

Yogurt and Fruit

**2 tablespoons plain yogurt
2 tablespoons pureed apricots,
applesauce, peaches or prunes**

Combine yogurt and pureed fruit; mix until well blended. Warm slightly before giving to baby. If the yogurt is ice cold warm the mixture slightly before giving to baby.

Yogurt, Fruit and Cottage Cheese

**1 tablespoon plain yogurt
1 tablespoon pureed banana,
pears, figs or dates
1 tablespoon cottage cheese**

Have ingredients at room temperature. Press fruit and cottage cheese through a baby food grinder and mix with yogurt until well blended.

Baked Apple and Raisins

**apples
raisins
butter, unsalted**

Core apples and fill center with raisins. Dot with butter. Put in baking pan with a little boiling water. Bake in a moderate oven for about 45 minutes or until tender.

After the apple has cooled, scoop out the raisins and cooked fruit and press through a baby food grinder.

Fruit-Juice Gelatin

1 teaspoon unflavored gelatin
1/3 cup fruit juice
1/2 cup pureed apricots, peaches,
  pears, berries or tropical fruit

Combine gelatin and fruit juice. Dissolve over hot water. Add pureed fruit. Before giving to baby chill the fruit and gelatin mixture until it becomes syrupy.

Banana Ice Cream

1 cup cream
2 small ripe bananas
1/4 teaspoon lemon juice

Whip cream until soft peaks form. Press bananas through a baby food grinder and stir in lemon juice. Combine whipped cream and bananas, mixing well. Pour into ice cube tray and freeze. Stir at regular intervals while the ice cream is freezing.

Fruit ice creams will soothe baby's gums when he is teething. If in season, try using 2 ripe persimmons in place of bananas. This will make a very tasty ice cream without adding any sweeteners.

Experiment with other ripe fruits or berries. Use 1/2 to 3/4 cup pureed fruit. Just be sure all fruit is thoroughly washed before pressing through a baby food grinder.

About La Leche League

La Leche League is a non-profit organization that gives helpful advice and encouragement to all mothers who want to breastfeed their babies. "La Leche," which is Spanish and is pronounced la lay-chay, means "The Milk."

There are approximately 2,800 La Leche League groups in 50 states in the United States and in 42 other countries. La Leche League now reaches more than a million persons each year through group meetings, correspondence, telephone conversations and League publications. The group leaders are capable of answering most problems concerned with the day-to-day nursing of infants.

League mothers do not give medical advice. However, the parent organization has a 34 member professional advisory board whose members are consulted on medical problems, evaluation of new research, and all material of a medical nature published by La Leche League International.

A mother who is interested in breastfeeding should write directly to the International headquarters to find out whether a League group exists in her area. If a group does not exist, La Leche League will correspond with you and/or give you information about the closest group. The League will give an information packet to anyone who writes to the following address:

La Leche League International, Inc.
9616 Minneapolis Avenue
Franklin Park, Illinois 60131

The League also publishes a book called *The Womanly Art of Breastfeeding*, which gives practical advice and encouragement to all mothers who want to breastfeed their babies. Besides the book, the League publishes a newsletter called "La Leche League News," which contains articles by doctors and practical hints and other news of interest to the nursing mother.

INDEX

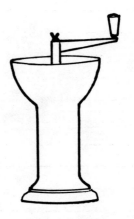

Diet Sheet

Favorite Recipes

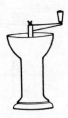

Favorite Recipes

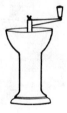

Favorite Recipes

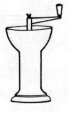

Favorite Recipes

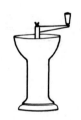

Notes

Notes

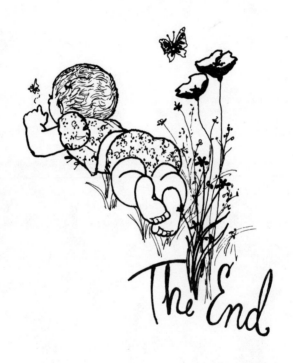

The End